This Notebook Belongs To:

詠春

"Wing Chun"

"Chi Sau in Wing Chun is to maintain one's flexibility and softness, all the while keeping in the strength to fight back, much like the flexible nature of bamboo" – Ip Man

ISBN: 9781072613350
Independently published
martialnotebooks@gmail.com

Date

Date

詠春

Date

Date

詠春

Date

Date

詠春

Date

Date

詠春

Date

Date

詠春

Date

Date

詠春

Date

Date

詠春

Date

Date

詠春

Date

Date

詠春

Date

Date

詠春

Date

Date

詠春

Date

Date

詠春

Date

Date

詠春

Date

Date

詠春

Date

Date

詠春

Date

Date

詠春

Date

Date

詠春

Date

Date

詠春

Date

Date

詠春

Date

Date

詠春

Date

Date

詠春

Date

Date

詠春

Date

Date

詠春

Date

Date

詠春

Date

Date

詠春

Date

Date

詠春

Date

Date

詠春

Date

Date

詠春

Date

Date

詠春

Date

Date

詠春

Date

Date

詠春

Date

Date

詠春

Date

Date

詠春

Date

Date

詠春

Date

Date

詠春

Date

Date

詠春

Date

Date

詠春

Date

Date

詠春

Date

Date

詠春

Date

Date

詠春

Date

Date

詠春

Date

Date

詠春

Date

Date

詠春

Date

Date

詠春

Date

Date

詠春

Date

Date

詠春

Date

Date

詠春

Date

Date

詠春

Date

Date

詠春

Date

www.ingramcontent.com/pod-product-compliance
Lightning Source LLC
Chambersburg PA
CBHW070433290526
45791CB00005B/1961
9781072613350